What we should all know about

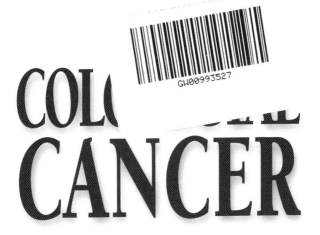

GW00993527

COL...

CANCER

What we should all know about Colorectal Cancer
Second edition

Written and edited under the auspices of

Dr David Cunningham
Head, Gastroenterology and Lymphoma Units,
The Royal Marsden Hospital NHS Trust, London

Contributors:

Dr Justin Waters
Specialist Registrar
The Royal Marsden Hospital NHS Trust, London

and

Mr Jon Tilsed
Consultant Colorectal Surgeon
Castle Hill Hospital
Hull and East Yorkshire NHS Trust, Hull

with

Heather Simmonds
and Fatima Patel
Mediscript Ltd

What we should all know about Colorectal Cancer
is published by

Mediscript
1 Mountview Court
310 Friern Barnet Lane
London N20 0LD
UK

ISBN 1-871211-58-1

First edition 2000

Contents

1 Introduction

Colorectal cancer is a disease of the large bowel, including the rectum (the final, pocket-like section of the bowel). It is something that many people do not want to talk about and may be unwilling to ask questions. If you or a member of your family has this disease, this book will help you understand what is happening.

The text first explains how cancer develops, and then how colorectal cancer develops. Current facts are given, showing how many people are affected, what the risk factors are, how the disease is diagnosed and the likelihood of a cure. Since surgery is usually involved in treatment, this is explained in some detail, with diagrams.

There are descriptions of typical cases, which may help you, and a section providing answers to some of the most commonly asked questions.

Information is also given on a wide variety of support groups, aiming to help patients and their families cope as well as possible with the condition.

This book aims to allow a clear understanding of colorectal cancer in a form that you can read at home in your own time. Most of what you read here may already be explained by your doctors or nurses, but this book will help you to clarify your knowledge and guide you towards asking them the most appropriate questions.

Various medical terms are explained fully in the text and a glossary of terms is also listed at the end of the book. Finally, an index is given for quick reference.

2 What is cancer?

Cancer develops as a result of an abnormal cell, which multiplies to produce millions of cells, forming a lump or tumour. The word 'tumour' simply means a swelling. If you have a tumour, you may be told that it is benign or else malignant. A diagnosis of malignancy at the primary tumour site is dependent on the expertise of the pathologist (a specialist in examining cells and tissues under a microscope). If your tumour is confirmed to be malignant, you will have a diagnosis of cancer.

This does not have to mean that you will die in the foreseeable future. Well over 200,000 people are diagnosed with cancer each year in the UK, and there are about 150,000 deaths, but this number appears to have been falling in recent years. Many cancers can be cured, especially when found in the early stages.

Unfortunately, cancer tends to spread out from its original site to surrounding tissues and to different parts of the body. This occurs when the primary (first-stage) cancer invades blood vessels and gets carried to other sites in the bloodstream and lymphatic system. New tumours may then be formed at distant sites and these are called secondary tumours or 'metastases'.

Cancers arise from disorders in genes

Genes are formed from deoxyribonucleic acid (DNA). A normal cell becomes cancerous when the genetic material (DNA) in the cell nucleus develops a malfunction and sends a signal that instructs the cell to divide and ignore any controlling signals from surrounding cells or hormones. This may occur in the body during an individual's lifetime (somatic change) or the malfunction may be inherited (hereditary defect). Although individual characteristics such as eye colour or height are the result of interactions from many different genes, molecular biologists are now beginning to identify the role of single genes in the steps that lead to cancer. It is, however, rare for any cancer to be caused by a single somatic mutation. In the case of colorectal cancer, several independent somatic mutations are required to produce a malignant cell. In contrast, with a hereditary defect, the potential for cancer is present at birth.

Effects at primary site

Growth of the tumour at its site of origin may produce some of the following symptoms:

◆ Obstruction (for example, blockage of the bowel due to bowel cancer)
◆ Other complications, such as bleeding, due to the growth spreading into blood vessels
◆ Loss of weight and loss of energy or appetite (sometimes)
◆ Pain (sometimes)
◆ Local swelling (not common)

3 What is colorectal cancer?

The colon and the rectum

Colorectal cancer means cancer (malignant swelling) in any part of the colon or rectum. This is a very large and important part of the human digestive system.

The colon and the rectum together form most of the large intestine or bowel. The intestine as a whole (large plus small) runs from the stomach to the anus, with the rectum forming a final collection pocket (see Figure 1, page 6). 'Anus' is the medical name for the opening through which waste matter (faeces) is discharged from the body. The bowel system also includes the caecum, a pouch between the small intestine and the colon sited just above the appendix. The small bowel carries only liquid and is excluded from the term 'colorectal'.

The left side of the colon is different from the right side because the colon has two basic functions, to allow food and water to be absorbed into the body and to act as a reservoir for the more solid waste. Thus, the contents of the right side (ascending colon) are fairly watery, while the contents of the left side (descending and sigmoid colon) and the rectum are more solid. Cancer arising on the right side of the colon may begin with vague abdominal aching, unlike the colic-type pain caused by obstructive left-side tumours.

How does colorectal cancer spread to become secondary cancer?

The spread of tumour cells from one organ to another can occur by direct invasion through the tissues or by the process of metastasis. Direct spreading of the tumour is relatively common with rectal cancer, because there are several organs very close to the rectum such as the bladder, the sacrum (part of the lower spine), the uterus and ovaries in women, and the prostate gland and seminal vesicles in men.

Metastasis means the spread of tumour cells via the lymphatic system (a network of vessels conveying lymph, a colourless fluid

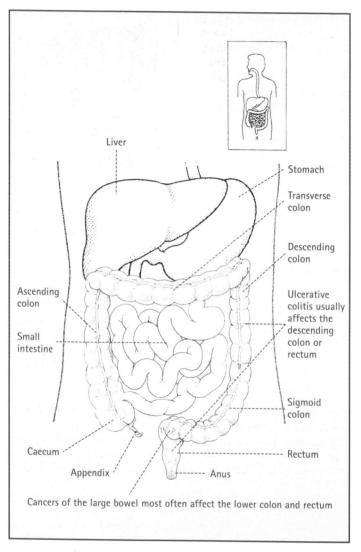

Liver

Stomach

Transverse colon

Descending colon

Ascending colon

Ulcerative colitis usually affects the descending colon or rectum

Small intestine

Sigmoid colon

Caecum

Rectum

Appendix

Anus

Cancers of the large bowel most often affect the lower colon and rectum

Figure 1: Diagram showing the colon and rectum, below the liver and the stomach. Inset also shows the gullet (throat), the food passage extending from the mouth to the stomach.

containing white blood cells) or via the blood stream. Cells are first released from the primary tumour to enter the circulation (lymph or blood), which carries them to distant parts of the body. The cells then become lodged in another organ, and begin to divide and grow to form a secondary tumour. Both colon and rectal cancers spread by metastasis. Sites commonly affected are the liver, lungs, bones and lymph nodes (small organs of the lymph system; Figure 2). Less commonly, secondaries may occur in the brain.

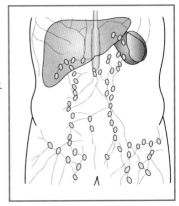

Figure 2: Part of the lymph node system (in the area of the colon) is shown as an example of this system.

How common is colorectal cancer?

In Western countries, colorectal cancer is one of the most common cancers and ranks second only to lung carcinoma as a cause of death from cancer. Tumours of the colon are slightly more frequent in women, while rectal tumours are slightly more common in men.

Age at onset

The risk of developing colorectal tumours begins to increase once men and women have passed the age of 30 years but only becomes high after the age of 50 years. People over 50 years of age make up only 37% of the population, but they account for 95% of cases of colorectal cancer. The average age at onset is 60–65 years for both sexes.

Early detection and prevention

Of all the major cancers, colorectal cancer is the most likely to be cured if the disease is identified sufficiently early and the best techniques are applied. At present, around 17,000 people die from colorectal cancer every year in England and Wales, or one death every 30 minutes. Up to 30,000 new cases are found annually, but many of these are not detected until the disease has advanced, and the prognosis (outlook) for patients with advanced colorectal cancer is still poor, despite new types of treatment. Therefore, prevention is very important (see Risks and causes), as is early detection (see Screening for colorectal cancer). When diagnosed at an early stage, 90% of colorectal cancer patients can be cured.

Colorectal cancer may begin with a change in bowel habits (more frequent, diarrhoea or constipation, or bleeding) or a vague abdominal aching. It is all too easy to ignore these small symptoms, thinking that they don't matter. You should always tell your doctor about any symptoms that last longer than two weeks, taking care to report how long the problem has been occurring and whether it is increasing. Small, benign growths may then be excised before they develop. Unfortunately, many people wait six to nine months before seeing a doctor and, at this stage, up to 50% may have a cancer that is very hard to cure, although palliative treatment to delay the growth of the cancer and improve the patient's quality of life will be worthwhile.

Risks and causes

The strongest risk factors are a history of chronic ulcerative colitis, a family history of colon cancer, especially familial adenomatous polyposis and hereditary non-polyposis colon cancer, and a previous history of colorectal adenomatous polyps.

Diets rich in fat and cholesterol have been linked to an increased risk of colorectal cancer. High levels of dietary protein, alcohol consumption and inactivity provide further risk. In contrast, a high intake of calcium, vegetables, fruit and fibre lowers the risk of this cancer.

Patients with inflammatory bowel disease (ulcerative colitis and Crohn's disease) are also more likely to develop colorectal cancer. The risk depends on how long the disease has lasted, the extent of colitis, the development of mucosal dysplasia (abnormal growth of the lining of the bowel wall) and on whether the symptoms have been continuous. If you have suffered from ulcerative colitis continuously for more than 20 years, you have a 30% risk of developing colorectal cancer. The risk is somewhat less if you have Crohn's disease.

A family history of colorectal cancer may be found in up to 15% of patients with this disease. Harmful genetic mutations are most likely to be observed in families in which the cancer is diagnosed at a young age (mean <40 years) and endometrial cancers are also present. (The endometrium is the membrane lining the womb.)

Screening for colorectal cancer

Treatment for colorectal cancer is most successful if the disease is discovered at an early stage. However, because it often causes no symptoms until it reaches a relatively advanced stage, some people have asked whether there is a test that could be used to detect early cancer. There are several difficulties with this approach.

First, a large number of people would need to be tested, most of whom would not have colorectal cancer, in order to discover the few people who are affected.

Second, none of the screening tests available (usually designed to detect minute traces of blood in the stools) are 100% accurate. This means that only one out of every 30-40 people whose screening test suggests that they have colorectal cancer, will, in fact, be affected. This naturally leads to considerable anxiety, as well as additional investigations that may carry a degree of risk to perform. Conversely, a few people whose screening test is negative, will actually have colorectal cancer, and will therefore be inappropriately reassured.

Currently, screening is only recommended for people who appear to have a particularly high risk of developing the disease. This includes those with close relatives who developed colorectal cancer at a young age, or those known to carry one of the rare genetic predispositions for the disease; people who have developed polyps or cancer previously; and people with inflammatory bowel disease (ulcerative colitis or Crohn's disease). The best method of screening this limited group of people is with regular colonoscopy, at intervals of between one and five years.

Signs and symptoms

The most common symptoms produced by colorectal cancer are bleeding from the rectum, a change in bowel habit and, sometimes, abdominal pain. However, these symptoms are much more often due to other, benign conditions such as haemorrhoids (piles) and the irritable bowel syndrome.

Colorectal cancer usually grows relatively slowly over a period of many months, and often only causes symptoms when it starts to cause a degree of blockage to the passage of faeces. This occurs earlier if the tumour is located towards the end of the bowel (sigmoid colon or rectum), where the faeces are more solid. About 60% of diagnosed colorectal cancers are in this area. Tumours in this region are more likely to cause visible bleeding from the rectum. The blood usually appears to streak the stool (faecal matter) surface or to be mixed in with the stool.

In contrast, tumours of the caecum and the ascending colon often do not produce any symptoms until they grow to a large size. Instead, they may be recognised because of the development of anaemia, which may be discovered from a blood test, or it may cause symptoms of tiredness and shortness of breath. Sometimes you can feel a mass or lump in the right side of the abdomen.

Diagnostic tests

None of these symptoms are specific for colorectal cancer. Therefore, you will need to undergo further, specialist investigations to confirm the diagnosis and plan your treatment.

Clinical examination may alert your doctor to suspicious features, such as signs of anaemia, the presence of a mass within the abdomen, or enlargement of other organs, such as the liver. The doctor will also examine your rectum to feel for a mass and to look for bleeding. To see the inside of the bowel, the doctor will normally use a sigmoidoscope (see Figure 3, page 12). This is a tube that is introduced into the lower part of the bowel via the anus,

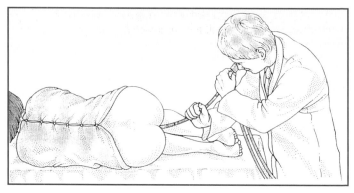

Figure 3: A doctor uses a sigmoidoscope to examine the inside lining of the lower part of the large bowel. Tissue samples can be taken for analysis.

which allows the doctor to examine the mucosa (inside lining) of the rectum and sigmoid colon, and take biopsies (tissue samples) of any abnormal areas. It may be somewhat uncomfortable but you will be able to go home immediately afterwards.

Examination of the colon

If there is any suspicion of colorectal cancer because of the symptoms or signs found, the rest of your bowel will be examined. There are two routine tests used to do this: barium enema and colonoscopy. You may need one or other of these tests, or even both.

Barium enema

This is an X-ray test of the bowel. Your bowel must be emptied before you come into the hospital (a laxative is used). At the hospital, a further washout of the bowel may be done by the insertion of liquid through a small tube. After you have passed this liquid down the toilet and your bowel is as clean as possible, a mixture of barium and air is inserted. This puts a contrast medium into the bowel to make it show up on the X-ray picture, and then X-rays are taken from several angles so that images of the whole large bowel from the anus to the caecum are obtained. Air is also blown into the bowel to improve the quality of the pictures, and thus improve the chances of detecting any abnormalities present.

Since you have to hold the barium mixture while the X-rays are taken, this test can be quite tiring and you may need a friend to go home with you. The test may cause constipation in the short term or the stools (waste material) may become white as the barium leaves your system.

Colonoscopy

This test uses a video endoscope on a flexible tube to look directly at the inside of the bowel. Your bowel must also be emptied before this examination, as for the barium enema. The tube is usually inserted into the bowel while you are under sedation. There is a camera mounted on the head of the tube so that the picture can be viewed on a TV screen.

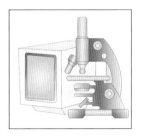

This method of examination is particularly useful because abnormal areas can be biopsied (sampled) and analysed to confirm the diagnosis. You will need an hour or two in hospital afterwards to recover from the sedation. Again, you may need someone to accompany you home. Colonoscopy does carry some risk of perforation, although this is very small.

Other diagnostic tests

Ultrasound scanning, computed tomography (CT) scanning and magnetic resonance imaging (MRI) are used to determine the extent of spread of colorectal cancer. MRI is particularly effective for assessing the local extent of rectal cancers, and is being used increasingly before treatment is started to guide the surgeon and oncologist as to the best way to proceed. These tests are quick and painless, with nothing inserted into your body.

CT scanning can reveal evidence of metastatic disease (secondary spread of cancer from its original site to other areas such as the liver or lungs). This is generally done as a routine test for all patients, either before or after surgery. It is also used to monitor patients' progress during treatment with chemotherapy or radiotherapy for metastatic disease.

What is a colonic polyp or adenoma?

Colorectal cancer develops gradually through several stages. A colonic polyp or adenoma is one of the early stages of this process. It is not a cancer in itself, but may develop into cancer with time. If polyps are discovered with the tests described above, they will be removed, usually at the time of colonoscopy. Repeat colonoscopic examinations will be recommended at intervals to make sure that no further polyps are developing.

Prognosis

Prognosis means forecast. The prognosis for your disease will tell you what you can expect in the future, how fast the disease is likely to develop and what are the chances of a cure. This will be an expert opinion but it is not a certainty. It is based on what has happened with other patients over a long period of time.

The prognosis of newly diagnosed colorectal cancer depends on the results of the investigations described above, and on the outcome of the initial treatment. Answers to the following questions are very important for a prognosis.

◆ Is the cancer confined to the bowel, or has it spread to other organs?

◆ Is an operation to remove the tumour possible and safe?

◆ Is the tumour completely blocking the bowel?

◆ Has the tumour perforated (broken through) the bowel wall?

The primary aim of treatment is to remove the cancer entirely with an operation, where this is possible. If this is successful the outlook can be very good, but there remains a risk that the cancer will recur. Careful examination of the specimen under the microscope will guide the surgeon and oncologist as to the degree of this risk, which will help them decide whether to recommend any additional treatment. The most important questions are as follows:

◆ Has the cancer been entirely removed, or are there cancer cells at the edge of the resected specimen?

◆ What is the degree of invasion of the cancer into the bowel wall?

◆ Are any lymph nodes within the specimen involved with the cancer?

◆ Are the small blood and lymph vessels within the tumour invaded by the cancer?

◆ How aggressive do the cancer cells appear?

5 Treatment

Cancer treatment aims to remove all clinical evidence of the disease, permanently if possible (curative treatment). If this cannot be done, your doctor aims to delay cancer growth and relieve your symptoms (palliative treatment). Thus, treatment for colorectal cancer can be divided into curative treatment for localised disease and palliative treatment for advanced or metastatic disease.

Curative treatment

Removal of all the cancer from the body by surgery is a pre-requisite for a cure, but is not always sufficient. This is because cancer cells that are too small to be seen by eye, or even by the most sensitive scans, may already have spread beyond the site of the primary tumour by the time it is removed. These cells can later give rise to secondary cancers. Additional treatment given after surgery can kill cancer cells that remain in the body, thus preventing them from developing into metastases. This is known as adjuvant treatment.

Palliative treatment

Palliative treatment is designed to control rather than cure the disease. It is considered successful if the patient's life is prolonged and the symptoms caused by the disease are lessened. An improvement in the quality of life is an important aim of this therapy.

Preoperative radiotherapy or chemoradiation

Preoperative treatment with radiotherapy (X-ray treatment) or chemoradiation (drugs plus X-rays) can sometimes shrink a rectal tumour down before surgery, so that the operation is easier to perform and more likely to be successful. If this is done, it may be possible for you to have an operation without having a colostomy (excision of part of the colon, directing the remaining end to an outlet at the front of the abdomen rather than the anus), which might be needed otherwise. With rectal tumours, preoperative radiotherapy reduces the risk of pelvic recurrence, which may lead to a longer life. The oncologists and surgeons will decide which is the best treatment for you, depending on the conditions of your cancer .

Surgery

Surgery has been the main treatment for colorectal cancer for over 100 years. It has undergone substantial advances during that time and new developments are being introduced continually. Surgery is now used for both prevention and treatment.

Removal of polyps

It has been known for many years that colorectal cancers develop from benign polyps. Not all polyps become malignant, but as there is no way of telling those that will become cancers from those that will not, they should all be removed. This can often be done through a flexible telescope (either flexible sigmoidoscopy or colonoscopy), allowing the polyps to be diagnosed and treated at the same time. This may be done under light sedation, but this is not always necessary.

Polyps with a 'stalk-like' base can usually be removed by passing a wire snare around the stalk like a lasso or noose (Figure 4). The polyp is then burnt off by passing an electric current through the stalk. This technique can also be used for polyps with a flat base. It is important that these polyps are checked microscopically to make sure that they do not contain areas of cancer. This usually takes a few days as the polyps have to be soaked for several hours in preservative, embedded in wax, cut into very thin slices and stained with special dyes before they are ready to be examined.

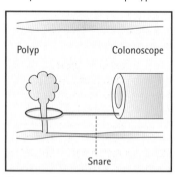

Figure 4: Colonoscopic polyp removal. The polyp is removed by using a snare, which is passed down a colonoscope.

Not all polyps are suitable for removal in this way. Large flat polyps or those known to contain areas of malignancy are usually best treated by other surgical procedures.

Transanal resection

Large rectal polyps can often be removed through an operating sigmoidoscope. This is essentially a metal tube that is inserted through the anus into the rectum under either a general or epidural anaesthetic and allows the surgeon to get to the polyp and remove it.

A recent advance on this technique is called transanal endoscopic microsurgery. This consists of a closed system in which the rectum is distended with carbon dioxide gas. Sealed ports (openings) in the endoscope are used to introduce operating instruments, while keeping the rectum distended. The system has binocular magnification to increase the surgeon's view so that not only can polyps be removed, but a complete segment of bowel can be cut out and the remaining ends sewn back together using this technique. This can be useful for large flat polyps and for early cancers in people who are too frail to undergo major surgery.

Familial adenomatous polyposis (FAP) and ulcerative colitis

People with FAP have a genetic abnormality that usually results in the growth of hundreds of colorectal polyps. If left, some of these would become malignant, giving rise to cancer at a young age. As it is not possible to remove all of these polyps individually, people with FAP will most often have all of the large bowel removed. This usually consists of removing the rectum and colon (procto-colectomy) together with the lining of the top of the anal canal (mucosectomy; see Figure 5, page 18).

People with extensive ulcerative colitis that has been present for many years are also at risk of developing bowel cancer. They will usually be kept on a programme of regular colonoscopic examinations at which random biopsies of the bowel lining are taken. If the biopsies show significant abnormalities (known as dysplasia), surgery will probably be recommended to prevent cancer developing. A number of surgical procedures may be performed. The colon is always removed, but the rectum may sometimes be left.

Removal of the rectum: forming a 'j pouch'

The rectum and anus together form an important functional unit that normally allows us to open our bowels when it is socially

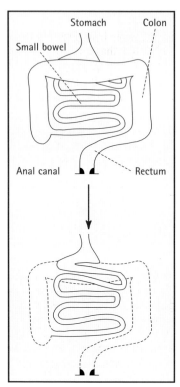

Figure 5: Proctocolectomy. Treatment for familial adenomatous polyposis (FAP) may involve removal of the upper part of the colon and rectum and also the lining (mucosa) of the upper part of the anal canal (a proctocolectomy with mucosectomy).

convenient. The rectum acts as a reservoir to reduce the number of bowel actions required and the anus usually remains tightly closed to prevent the contents of the rectum from leaking out.

If the rectum is removed, some of the reservoir function will be lost. This may result in more frequent bowel actions. Over a period of time the colon can adapt and take over some of this function. This adaptation is usually most noticeable during the first year after surgery. People who have had both colon and rectum removed (a proctocolectomy) would almost certainly have diarrhoea if the small bowel were joined directly onto the anal canal. To overcome this problem, a reservoir can be created out of the small bowel by forming a pouch. This is usually done by folding the end of the small bowel back on itself in the shape of a 'j', joining the adjacent limbs of the loop together with two lines of stitches and then dividing the bowel between the lines to create a j pouch (Figure 6). The base of the j is then opened and joined onto the anal canal. Although pouches were originally hand-sewn, they are usually formed now by using a number of stapling devices.

Figure 6: Construction of a j pouch. (a) A small bowel pouch can be made by folding the cut end back on itself to form a j. (b) Viewed from above at level X–Y. (c) A reservoir is made by joining the two pieces of bowel together with two lines of stitches and cutting the bowel between the joins. (d) The base of the j is then opened and joined to the anal canal.

A pouch will not work as well as a normal rectum. Most surgeons would consider four to six bowel actions a day with a pouch as a good result. The motions are also looser than those produced from a normal bowel. Good anal sphincter function (the sphincter is the ring of muscle that guards the opening and allows you to evacuate the rectum or hold the contents in at will) is essential to prevent incontinence and, as a result, a pouch is not suitable for everyone who has had a proctocolectomy. For this reason pouches tend to be reserved for younger people with good sphincter function. Removing the colon and rectum and restoring bowel continuity with a pouch is known as a restorative proctocolectomy. This (together with a mucosectomy) is the usual operation performed for FAP, and it can also be performed for cancer prevention in ulcerative colitis.

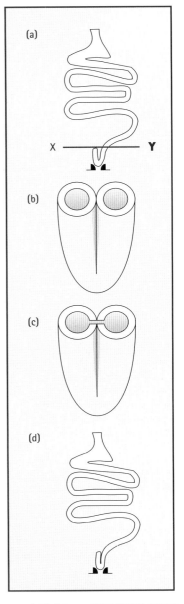

Ulcerative colitis: ileorectal anastomosis

In people with ulcerative colitis, an alternative to the 'j' pouch is to remove the colon and join the small bowel to the rectum (an ileorectal anastomosis; Figure 7). This preserves some of the reservoir function of the rectum and is usually better than a pouch. However, the bowel motions will still be looser than normal and there will still be a risk of developing cancer of the rectum in the future. This risk is small, but if you have had a colectomy for extensive ulcerative colitis that has been present for many years you should undergo regular examinations. As the rectum is usually less than 15 cm long, it is much easier to examine than the colon. If dysplasia or malignancy develops, the rectum should be removed. This is called a proctectomy.

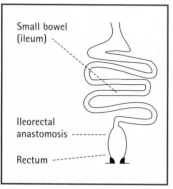

Figure 7: Ileorectal anastomosis.

Small bowel (ileum)

Ileorectal anastomosis

Rectum

Ulcerative colitis: ileostomy

An alternative to colectomy and ileorectal anastomosis or restorative proctocolectomy is to remove the colon and rectum and bring out the small bowel onto the front of the abdomen to form an ileostomy. When this is done the anal canal will also be removed and the resulting hole will be sewn up (Figure 8). This is a panproctocolectomy. It has the advantage of eliminating all risk of bowel cancer and avoiding debilitating bowel frequency and incontinence. A bag is worn on the front of the abdomen to collect waste (an ileostomy bag).

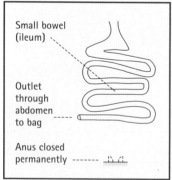

Small bowel (ileum)

Outlet through abdomen to bag

Anus closed permanently

Figure 8: Panproctocolectomy. The colon, rectum and anus are removed. The small bowel is brought out into the abdomen as an ileostomy and the hole where the anus was is closed.

Surgical treatment for colorectal cancer

Colorectal cancer develops from the inner lining of the bowel (the mucosa) and may spread directly through the bowel wall into neighbouring layers or structures. It may also spread through lymphatic channels to involve local lymph glands (now known as lymph nodes; see Figure 2, page 7). These microscopic channels pass alongside the blood vessels supplying the bowel. Bowel cancers that have spread to these lymph nodes are still potentially curable. As a result, most operations for colorectal cancer involve removing the segment of bowel containing the tumour with a margin of healthy tissue on either side of it, together with the major blood vessels supplying it.

Curative procedures for colon cancer

The precise operation for cancer of the colon or rectum will depend on the location of the tumour (Figure 9). In addition to removing the affected colon and its blood supply, a curative operation aims to restore bowel continuity by joining the two remaining ends together. For various reasons joining colon (or large bowel) to the small bowel (ileocolic anastomosis) tends to heal better than joining it to colon (colocolic anastomosis). A surgeon will weigh the benefits of an ileocolic anastomosis against the effects of removing

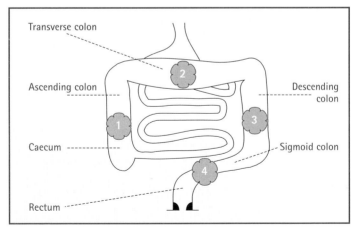

Figure 9: The surgical procedure that will be applied depends on the location of the tumour.

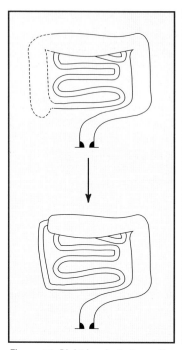

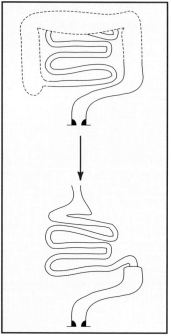

Figure 10: Right hemicolectomy. The right side of the colon is removed and the small bowel is joined to the remaining colon.

Figure 11: Extended right hemi-colectomy. The right side of the colon is removed in continuity with a variable amount of colon that can extend as far as the sigmoid colon. The small bowel is joined to the remaining colon.

more colon. For this reason, tumours of the caecum and ascending colon (position 1 in Figure 9) will be treated by a right hemi-colectomy (Figure 10) while tumours of the transverse (position 2 in Figure 9) and descending colon (position 3 in Figure 9) may be treated by an extended right hemicolectomy (Figure 11).

Tumours of the sigmoid colon may be removed with part of the rectum and this procedure is known as an anterior resection (as the rectum is approached from the front; Figure 12). However, the surgeon may decide to remove only the part of the colon

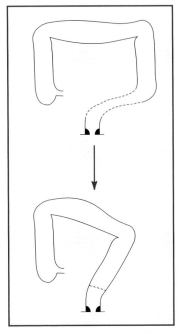

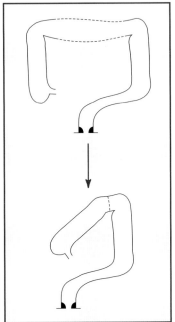

Figure 12: Anterior resection. The sigmoid colon and upper part of the rectum are removed and the colon is joined to the remaining rectum.

Figure 13: Transverse colectomy. The transverse colon is removed and the two remaining ends of colon are joined.

containing the tumour and this is known as a segmental resection. Tumour 2 (Figure 9, page 21) might be treated by removing the transverse colon (a transverse colectomy; Figure 13), tumour 3 (Figure 9) by a left hemicolectomy (Figure 14, page 24) and tumour 4 (Figure 9) by a sigmoid colectomy (Figure 15, page 24).

Curative surgery for cancer of the rectum

Gaining access to the colon is relatively straightforward. A cut is made through the front of the abdomen and this can be enlarged to provide a space big enough for the surgical team to work. However, getting to the rectum can be difficult. It lies inside the pelvis, which forms a rigid ring of bone through which the surgical team has to operate. The tumour is usually approached through the

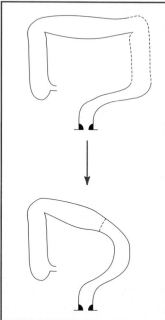

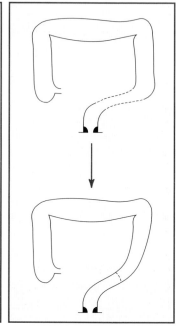

Figure 14: Left hemicolectomy. The left half of the colon is removed and the two remaining ends of colon are joined.

Figure 15: Sigmoid colectomy. The sigmoid colon is removed and the remaining colon and rectum are joined.

abdomen and removed by an anterior resection (Figure 12). The larger the tumour, the lower the tumour and the narrower the pelvis, the more difficult it becomes to remove the tumour from above and to join the remaining bowel ends together. The female pelvis, having evolved for childbirth, is usually much wider than the male, but even in women, anterior resection is not always possible.

When it is not possible to remove the tumour and a margin of healthy tissue from above, a combined approach from above and below is used. This is called an abdominoperineal excision of the rectum (and is usually known as an 'APER', an 'APE' or an 'APR'). One cut is made through the abdomen and another is made around the anus (in the perineum). The anal canal and rectum are removed and the hole produced in the perineum is closed. In this operation the

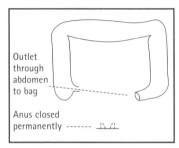

Outlet
through
abdomen
to bag

Anus closed
permanently

Figure 16: Abdominoperineal excision of the rectum (APER). The rectum and anus are removed. The colon is brought out onto the abdomen as a colostomy, and the hole where the anus has been removed is closed.

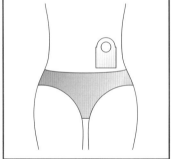

Figure 17: Colostomy. The colon is brought out onto the abdomen and drains into a disposable bag that is stuck onto the skin over the stoma or outlet (see page 26).

colon is brought out onto the skin through the abdomen to form a colostomy (Figures 16 and 17).

In recent years, there have been a number of important developments in the treatment of rectal cancer. Surgeons can now pass a stapling device through the anus to join colon and rectum where it would not be possible to sew them together from above. As a result, most rectal tumours can now be treated by anterior resection, whereas in the past nearly all would have required APER with a permanent colostomy.

Total mesorectal excision

As mentioned before, the bowel's lymphatic vessels form a route along which malignant cells can spread. These paths from the colon are well defined as they pass with the blood supply along an easily identifiable sheet of tissue called the mesentery. This can be seen coming off the bowel like the sail of a boat coming off its mast.

In contrast, the mesentery of the rectum forms a tube around it, something like the pastry of a sausage roll. This is called the mesorectum, and it is important that the tumour-bearing rectum is removed together with the mesorectum as a single package of tissue. For lower rectal tumours, the whole of the mesorectum should be removed. This technique is known as total mesorectal excision. It has been shown to reduce the rate of tumour recurrence significantly and is currently being adopted by the surgical community.

Locally invasive disease

Colorectal cancer may grow into neighbouring tissues, such as the muscle of the abdomen, loops of bowel, or stomach, and the tumour extension can usually be removed in one piece with the bowel (an 'en bloc' resection). This can often provide a cure.

It may be useful for the surgeon to assess a rectal tumour by performing an examination under anaesthetic and to arrange appropriate scans to see whether or not local invasion has occurred. Direct spread of tumour into the womb can be treated by removing it (en bloc hysterectomy) together with the rectum. If other structures are involved in rectal cancer, a course of radiotherapy might be suggested to shrink the tumour before surgery is performed.

Stomas

The word 'stoma' is derived from the Greek word meaning a 'mouth' or 'opening'. In the context of bowel surgery, it is used to describe the artificial opening produced when a piece of bowel is brought out onto the skin of the abdomen. The bowel contents are drained through the stoma into a disposable bag that is stuck onto the skin over the stoma (see Figure 17, page 25). There are two main types of stoma: an ileostomy (where the opening is made into the small bowel) and a colostomy (where it is made into the colon). Stomas may be permanent or temporary. For example, a permanent colostomy will be formed after an APER because the operation produces only one end of bowel and there is nowhere else for it to go. A temporary stoma may be formed to allow time for the join between two ends of bowel to heal. This is particularly likely for low rectal cancers. The join can be checked by putting an appropriate dye into the bowel and taking X-rays of it. If there is no leak, the stoma can usually be reversed.

Hartmann's procedure

Sometimes, the first time someone with bowel cancer is aware of a problem is when the bowel blocks or bursts. There will usually have been some symptoms that have been ignored or else not recognised. If this has happened, emergency surgery may be needed and, under these circumstances, the surgeon may not consider it safe to rejoin the bowel ends once the tumour has been removed. Both ends of the bowel may be brought out as a stoma, or in the case of a tumour in the sigmoid colon or rectum, the remaining rectum may be closed and left inside the abdomen. This is known as a Hartmann's procedure (Figure 18). The two ends of bowel can be joined together at a later date when a full recovery from the first operation has been made.

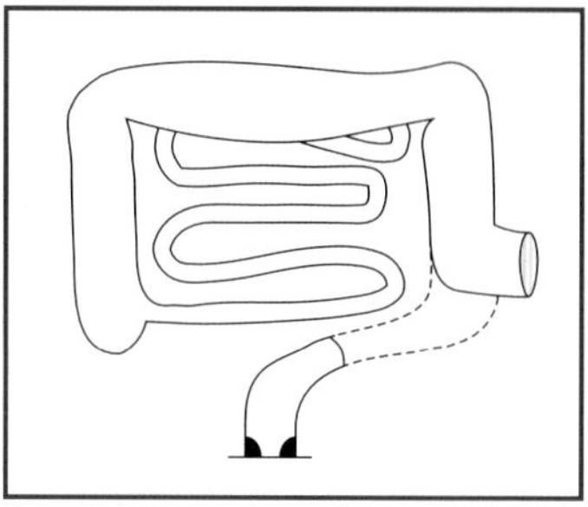

Figure 18: Hartmann's procedure. Part of the sigmoid colon (or rectum) is removed. One end is brought out as a colostomy, while the other end is closed and left inside the abdomen.

Surgery for metastatic disease

Bowel cancer may also spread through the bloodstream to form distant metastases. These most commonly affect the liver. Under certain conditions, it may be possible to remove part of the liver containing metastases. This is a major undertaking but, in suitable selected cases, about a third of those having liver surgery will be cured. Similar results have been reported for surgery when the cancer has spread to the lung.

Future surgical developments

A number of centres are currently developing techniques of anorectal reconstruction to avoid a permanent colostomy. For example, the colon can be brought out onto the perineum in place of a removed anus and an artificial sphincter can be created around this from one of the thigh muscles. This 'sphincter' can be switched on and off by remote control through a small 'pacemaker' device concealed under the skin. A completely 'self-contained' artificial sphincter can also be used for this purpose. However, these procedures are still being developed and, as a result, are not widely available.

Adjuvant treatment

Adjuvant treatment is additional treatment given after surgery, in order to kill any remaining cancer cells in the body.

Adjuvant chemotherapy

Chemotherapy means treatment with drugs and is used as an adjuvant to prevent the recurrence of colorectal cancer after successful surgery. It is known to benefit some groups of patients, notably those who have lymph node involvement with cancer, and also those who have tumours that extend through the bowel wall.

The standard treatment is with the drugs 5-fluorouracil (5-FU) and leucovorin (also known as folinic acid), given for six months in total. This can cause some side effects, including mouth ulcers, diarrhoea, fatigue and reddening of the skin of the hands and feet (see Tables 1 and 2, pages 30 and 31). Nausea and significant hair loss are uncommon.

This treatment is usually administered as a daily injection for five consecutive days every four to five weeks, but other schedules are also in use. For instance, 5-fluorouracil can be given as a continuous infusion by a portable infusion pump, carried by the patient. This method may be more effective at killing cancer cells, and you may suffer less from side effects.

In women, suppression of the ovaries by chemotherapy may mean that menstrual periods disappear during treatment. Often, they come back, but for women in their late 30s and 40s, menopause may occur early. Chemotherapy can also cause abnormalities in children conceived during and after treatment. Therefore, fertile women will need to use contraception while undergoing chemotherapy and for at least one year afterwards.

Some newer drugs are being investigated as adjuvant treatment, but these are currently used for colorectal cancer only within clinical trials.

Adjuvant radiotherapy

Rectal cancer is often treated with radiotherapy in addition to surgery. Radiotherapy is an X-ray treatment that can kill cancer cells within the field of treatment (the area that the X-rays are focused on). Due to its location deep in the pelvis, and the close proximity of other structures and organs, rectal cancer has a tendency to recur at the same site from which it was initially removed (known as local recurrence). Radiotherapy to this area reduces the risk of local recurrence, hopefully avoiding some of the more severe symptoms that rectal cancer can produce.

Radiotherapy may be given either before or after surgery, and may last anything from five days to several weeks. Individual treatments (fractions) are usually given on a daily basis from Monday to Friday. Side effects of radiotherapy are tiredness, soreness of the skin in the region being treated and, occasionally, diarrhoea or a discharge from the rectum. Chemotherapy and radiotherapy can also be given together (known as chemoradiation). This may be more effective in preventing both local recurrence and metastatic disease.

Treatment of advanced colorectal cancer

Advanced colorectal cancer is disease that has spread from its original location in the bowel wall to other sites in the body. This may be present when the disease is first diagnosed, or may be caused by a recurrence of the disease. Treatment with chemotherapy can be effective in controlling the symptoms of advanced colorectal cancer, and also prolongs the life of some patients. However, chemotherapy does not cure this disease. If you are in this situation, the treatment selected for you is a balance between the possible benefit you may gain from it and the side effects that it may cause. Radiotherapy can also be used in some circumstances to control symptoms. For instance, pain resulting from bone metastases can be effectively treated with a short course of radiotherapy to the area affected.

Chemotherapy

For around 40 years, the standard treatment was with 5-fluorouracil and leucovorin (see Adjuvant treatment). Delivery of these drugs by intravenous infusion (direct delivery into a vein) is becoming more widely practised, but a number of different schedules are used in different hospitals (see Table 1, page 30). Of all patients treated in this way, roughly 20% to 30% will achieve a reduction in the size of their tumours, and for the same number again, the disease will be stable for a period of time.

Other drug regimens have also been used successfully (see Table 1, page 30). Some of these will probably be used more commonly in the future, as the results of clinical trials indicate that they are more effective at shrinking disease, and prolong life in more patients while maintaining the quality of their life.

The obvious drawback of using more drugs is that the number of side effects may be increased. To some extent, the type of

> *Table 1: Drug regimens used in advanced colorectal cancer*
>
> ◆ 5-Fluorouracil + leucovorin by daily injection for 5 days every 4 weeks
> ◆ 5-Fluorouracil + leucovorin by weekly injection
> ◆ Irinotecan combined with 5-fluorouracil + leucovorin (several schedules)
> ◆ Irinotecan by 2- or 3-weekly injection
> ◆ Continuous infusion of 5-fluorouracil
> ◆ Continuous infusion of 5-fluorouracil + mitomycin C
> ◆ Weekly 24-hour infusion of 5-fluorouracil + leucovorin
> ◆ Fortnightly 48-hour infusion of 5-fluorouracil + leucovorin
> ◆ Oxaliplatin combined with 5-fluorouracil + leucovorin (several schedules)
> ◆ Capecitabine tablets daily for 2 of every 3 weeks
> ◆ Uracil/ftorafur (UFT) plus oral leucovorin tablets daily for 4 of every 5 weeks

chemotherapy recommended for you will depend on your general fitness, because less fit patients are more likely to suffer severe side effects. Some of the latest drugs have predictable, manageable and non-cumulative side effects.

Regional chemotherapy

An alternative approach to giving chemotherapy systemically by intravenous administration or by mouth, is to give the chemotherapy directly into the affected organ. This is called regional chemotherapy, and is generally applied to liver metastases. The drugs are injected into a blood vessel that supplies the liver, which produces a high concentration of the drug at the site of the cancer.

Laser therapy and focused ultrasound therapy

Liver metastases are the most common and can be treated with laser therapy; investigators are currently developing focused

> **Table 2: Common side effects of chemotherapy drugs frequently used in colorectal cancer**
>
> **5-Fluorouracil**
> - Mouth ulcers
> - Diarrhoea
> - Red and sore hands and feet
> - Increased susceptibility to infection
>
> **Irinotecan**
> - Diarrhoea
> - Increased susceptibility to infection
> - Lethargy
> - Nausea and vomiting
>
> **Oxaliplatin**
> - Diarrhoea
> - Increased susceptibility to infection
> - Pins and needles, numbness and other unusual sensations that could be irreversible
> - Nausea and vomiting
> - Anaemia
>
> **Raltitrexed**
> - Diarrhoea
> - Lethargy
> - Increased susceptibility to infection
>
> **Mitomycin C**
> - Nausea and vomiting
> - Reduced platelet count (bleeding and bruising)

ultrasound for this purpose. Both these techniques rely on the generation of heat within the tumour to kill the cancer cells.

Metastasectomy

In some people, secondary tumours can be removed entirely with an operation called metastasectomy. Surgery is usually recommended only if a single organ is affected (usually the lung or liver). See also Surgery for metastatic disease (page 27). The chance of success depends on the exact location of the secondary tumour or tumours within the organ, and the fitness of the patient for major surgery.

Chemotherapy is often given as well to try to eradicate any other microscopic tumour deposits that may be present. Some patients treated in this way do appear to be cured of their disease.

6 Management of the side effects associated with treatment

The chemotherapy drugs used to treat colorectal cancer can cause some side effects (see Table 2, page 31). Different drugs tend to be associated with specific types of side effect, but some are common to most of the drugs.

Fatigue

Radiotherapy, chemotherapy and colorectal cancer itself can cause fatigue. Sometimes this is the result of anaemia (see Red blood cells on page 34), which can be corrected by blood transfusion. However, more commonly, no specific treatable cause can be found. This can be a particularly difficult and frustrating side effect, as it often limits the amount of normal activity a patient can manage.

Nausea and vomiting

Although many people think nausea and vomiting are common side effects of chemotherapy, this is no longer the case. Some chemotherapy drugs, including 5-fluorouracil, rarely cause any significant nausea or vomiting.

For other drugs that are more likely to cause these side effects, very effective anti-sickness drugs are now available that prevent nausea and vomiting in most people. You may be given an anti-sickness injection just before you begin chemotherapy, and anti-sickness tablets to take at home for the first two or three days. Symptoms after this time are unusual. Different types of anti-sickness drugs can be used in the rare cases where the initial treatment fails to control the symptoms adequately.

Hair loss

Hair loss is very unusual with most of the drugs used to treat colorectal cancer. If this does occur, a wig should be provided through the health service.

Haematological complications

These are complications of the blood. Most chemotherapy drugs can reduce the ability of the bone marrow to produce normal blood cells. Three different types of cell can be affected: the white blood cells, the red blood cells and the platelets.

White blood cells

These help your body to fight infection. If they are depleted by chemotherapy, you may be at risk from serious infection by bacteria, which is life-threatening if not properly and promptly treated. You and your doctor should be aware of the need for expert diagnosis and treatment if you become suddenly unwell while receiving chemotherapy.

Red blood cells

These carry oxygen to the tissues and organs of the body. Depletion of these cells results in anaemia (see Fatigue on page 33). This is not usually a serious side effect, and can be corrected by blood transfusion or erythropoietin preparations.

Platelets

Platelets help to prevent bleeding and bruising. When they are depleted, the patient may notice bruises appearing spontaneously, or bleeding from the gums or nose. If this happens, tell your doctor, as a transfusion of platelets may be necessary.

Diarrhoea

This is a relatively common side effect of several of the chemotherapy drugs used in colorectal cancer. If it is severe and prolonged, diarrhoea can lead to dehydration, and even death. If you are suffering from diarrhoea, you must make sure that you drink enough water. If you are unable to drink adequately, fluids may have to be administered intravenously via a drip. Antidiarrhoeal tablets will also be prescribed for you to start taking as soon as you first develop diarrhoea. However, you must ask your consultant or specialist for advice if the diarrhoea persists for more than 24 hours.

7 Complications of colorectal cancer

Bowel obstruction

The symptoms of bowel obstruction are nausea and vomiting, abdominal pain and swelling, and constipation. This can occur as a result of a primary tumour blocking the bowel, before surgery is performed to remove it. Bowel obstruction can also result from adhesions. These are fibrous bands that form in the abdomen after surgery, as a reaction to the process of surgery itself. A third cause is recurrence of the cancer within the abdomen. This can produce an inflammatory reaction on the surface of the tissues lining the abdomen (known as the peritoneum), blocking the bowel from the outside.

Bowel obstruction can sometimes be treated by resting the bowel. This means that you will not be able to eat or drink and, instead, you will be given fluid intravenously. A very narrow tube is also passed down the throat into the stomach, to empty the stomach contents, and prevent you from vomiting. Drugs may be used to reduce the swelling of the bowel wall. If these measures are unsuccessful, an operation may be required to relieve the obstruction.

Ascites

Ascites is excessive fluid that collects within the abdomen, which can lead to uncomfortable abdominal swelling. It is caused by secondary colorectal cancer involving the abdominal linings (peritoneum).

It can be treated by draining the fluid from the abdomen with a soft plastic tube, which is inserted after the skin is numbed by local anaesthetic. Sometimes, chemotherapy drugs are introduced into the abdominal cavity to try to shrink down the peritoneal tumours, and slow down the collection of fluid.

Jaundice

Jaundice is a yellow colour of the skin and eyes that results from liver damage, or blockage of the normal drainage of bile from the liver. This can be produced by metastatic colorectal cancer involving the liver, or the lymph nodes near the liver.

It can sometimes be relieved by putting a stent (plastic tube) in the bile duct, across the area of blockage. If this is not possible, drugs can be used to relieve itching, which is the main symptom of this type of jaundice. Chemotherapy treatment can improve jaundice if it shrinks the tumour in and around the liver.

Shortness of breath and coughing

These two symptoms can be produced by metastatic colorectal cancer involving the lungs. This may either be due to accumulation of fluid around the lungs (pleural effusion), or to destruction of the lung tissue (infiltration).

Breathlessness resulting from a pleural effusion can be relieved by drainage of the fluid by a needle inserted between the ribs, or through a soft plastic tube. Sometimes a chemotherapy drug is put into the pleural cavity (the space around the lungs) to prevent further accumulation of fluid. Systemic chemotherapy treatment can improve these symptoms if it effectively shrinks the metastatic disease.

Bone secondaries

If metastatic colorectal cancer affects your bones, they may be painful. This can usually be treated with painkillers and local radiotherapy. Sometimes the bones involved threaten to break, and an orthopaedic operation may be required to strengthen the area.

Nerve damage

Another source of pain from metastatic colorectal cancer is pressure on nerve fibres. The pattern of pain often follows the course of the nerve affected. For instance, pressure on nerves within the pelvis can produce pain that shoots down the leg. Radiotherapy to the tumour can often produce rapid relief of this symptom, and painkillers can also be effective.

Sometimes, pressure on nerves can cause weakness of the legs or arms, or if the spinal cord is affected, can cause paralysis and affect bladder or bowel function. This requires urgent treatment with steroids and radiotherapy, after which a certain degree of recovery is possible.

Fatigue and weight loss

Fatigue and weight loss often occur as temporary reactions to chemotherapy, but can also be caused by advanced colorectal cancer. Chemotherapy treatment may be effective in improving these symptoms. You may be given nutritional supplements to keep up your body weight and energy levels.

What we should all know about colorectal cancer

Adjusting to the diagnosis and primary treatment

Most people feel very anxious and depressed after a diagnosis of cancer, especially younger people and those with previous psychological difficulties. However, 95% of colorectal cancer patients are over the age of 50 years. It seems that about 30% of patients at least need specific counselling, preferably from someone with special training. Many others will benefit from such counselling. Or you may simply find it useful and comforting to be able to share your experiences with other people who are in a similar predicament.

You should not hold back, therefore, from seeking whatever help is available (see Support groups and counselling). Remember, there is simply no substitute for careful counselling. You may, for example, have others dependent on you.

It has also become clear from research that the patient's attitude to cancer and its treatment is profoundly influenced by the first consultation when the diagnosis is made. Therefore your doctor may suggest that your partner, a member of your family or a close friend go with you on your visits to the specialist. This can help to lessen your feelings of isolation. A supportive companion can also help you to remember details about the prognosis and treatment that you may misunderstand or forget in the shock of learning about your disease. You may need to read parts of this book a number of times.

All the treatments discussed in this book are traumatic in different ways. This means that, both mentally and physically, you will be going through a very tough time, sometimes over a period of many months before your treatment is completed. There will also be uncertainty about its success for many more months.

Your emotions and reactions

Even with the best support, you may need a long time to accept the situation. Anger, shock and even denial are normal reactions to bad news. It is hardly surprising, therefore, that any cancer is a challenge not only to the patient, but also to family, friends and professional carers.

Management of a colostomy

Many dedicated volunteers in support groups are available to help you (see Support Groups and Counselling). These are living proof that life can carry on as normal after a colostomy, that self-esteem returns and that involvement in home, work and recreational activity can continue just as before.

Problems of advanced disease and terminal illness

An accurate appraisal of the prognosis requires expert knowledge and may require careful investigation of the stage of disease to provide the necessary information if you really wish to know how the disease is likely to progress.

For some patients, denial of the prognosis may be a reasonable and effective way of coping with the situation.

When the news is bad, sharing information may be a gradual process: a trained and sensitive carer will recognise how much you want to know at any given time.

Although patients with advanced colorectal cancer have a fatal disorder, life may be prolonged by some treatments. This may allow time for you and your family to become reconciled to your illness.

9 Patient profiles

Introduction

When you have a serious illness, it often helps to learn what happened to others in a similar situation. The profiles given below are of patients whose colorectal cancer followed a typical course, with treatment outcomes that are very commonly observed. This may give you some idea of what to expect.

Name   Edward
Age   72

Edward went to his doctor complaining of increasing constipation and occasional abdominal pain. His doctor arranged for him to have a barium enema, which showed a stricture in the sigmoid colon. He was referred to a specialist colorectal surgeon who performed a sigmoidoscopy. This confirmed that a tumour growth was narrowing the sigmoid colon, and a biopsy showed that the tumour was malignant.

Edward then had an operation to remove the tumour, which was successful, and the bowel was joined up without the need for a colostomy. When the pathologist examined the material that had been removed, he found that the tumour had been completely excised, and confined to the bowel wall with no involvement of lymph nodes. There were no other adverse features present. A CT scan showed no evidence of tumour spread.

No additional treatment was recommended for Edward, and he remains well three years later, with no evidence of active disease.

Name   Edith
Age   66

Edith had been becoming increasingly tired and short of breath over the course of several months. One day she felt a lump in the right side of her abdomen. She went to the doctor who did some blood tests and referred her to a gastroenterologist who arranged a colonoscopy. The blood tests showed that she was anaemic, and the colonoscopy revealed a tumour of the caecum. A biopsy showed this to be malignant.

She underwent an operation, which was successful in removing the tumour. Pathological examination showed lymph node involvement, and the tumour cells were of an aggressive type, but a CT scan showed no further disease. Adjuvant chemotherapy was therefore recommended, and she continued this for six months. Initially, she had some side effects, comprising mouth ulcers and diarrhoea, but these improved after a minor adjustment in her chemotherapy dosage.

She began to feel rather tired towards the end of treatment, but after the chemotherapy finished, she was able to get back to normal. She had a further routine CT scan a year later that showed no evidence of relapse, and she continues to remain well.

Name   Martin
Age   55

Martin noticed some blood in his motions and went to his GP. She found a mass in his rectum, and referred him immediately to a colorectal surgeon. A biopsy of the mass showed that it was a malignant tumour of the rectum and a CT scan was arranged. This showed that the tumour was inoperable, due to invasion into surrounding structures, and Martin was therefore referred to an oncologist.

Treatment with a combination of chemotherapy and radiotherapy was recommended. The chemotherapy was given as a continuous infusion of 5-fluorouracil through a Hickman line, with additional injections of mitomycin C.

At the end of three months of treatment, a CT scan was repeated. This showed a very good response and the tumour was now felt to be operable. To confirm this impression, an MRI scan was performed of the pelvic area, and the result of this was in favour of an operation.

The tumour was then resected. This was achieved without the need for a permanent colostomy, although a temporary colostomy was required to protect the join of the two ends of the bowel. The pathology showed that active tumour was present in the specimen, and lymph nodes were involved, but the tumour had been completely removed.

A further three months of chemotherapy was given, and since then, Martin has remained well.

Name Mary
Age   35

Mary has a family history of colorectal cancer, her father having been diagnosed with the disease at the age of 30. She undergoes regular screening colonoscopy, and has had a number of polyps removed from her colon in the past. At the latest colonoscopy, a more extensive tumour was detected, and the biopsy revealed this to contain an invasive cancer. She therefore had an operation to remove the tumour. The pathology showed that this tumour was at a very early stage, only involving the inner lining of the bowel (the mucosa), and not invading the muscle layers of the bowel wall. There was also no evidence of tumour cells in any lymph nodes. No further treatment was recommended, but Mary continues to have regular screening colonoscopy.

Name Bill
Age   74

Bill developed increasing abdominal pain after being very constipated for several weeks. He was taken by ambulance to the Accident and Emergency Department, where bowel obstruction was diagnosed. An emergency gastrograffin (a contrast medium, like barium) enema showed an obstruction low in the rectum. Bill required an operation without delay to relieve the obstruction. A large tumour was found to be causing the blockage. This was removed, but because of the size and position of the tumour, a colostomy was necessary. The surgeon also examined Bill's liver, and unfortunately found several secondary tumours there. Both the primary tumour specimen and biopsies of the liver metastases were confirmed to be the same type of cancer, originating in the rectum.

Bill made a very good recovery from the operation, and was referred to an oncologist for consideration of further treatment. After discussion of the possible side effects, he decided to have treatment, which consisted of a 5-FU infusion, given via a Hickman line. During this treatment, Bill developed slight reddening and soreness of his hands, and his fingernails became discoloured and brittle, but he had no other problems. CT scans performed at intervals through his treatment showed a reduction in the size of the tumours in the liver, and treatment was stopped after six months. After that, Bill continued to have check-ups every three months but, seven months later, he started getting pain in his right leg. A further CT scan showed a local recurrence of the rectal cancer that was pressing on the nerves supplying the leg, and regrowth of the liver metastases. He was treated with a course of radiotherapy to the pelvic area, which dramatically improved his symptoms. He remained relatively fit and active, and was therefore offered further chemotherapy, this time with a different drug, irinotecan. This caused hair loss, and Bill felt quite tired for a week or so after each chemotherapy injection. However, for the other two weeks he was quite well.

He has now finished his third course of chemotherapy, and another CT scan has shown that his liver tumours have begun to shrink again.

Name   Pauline
Age   61

Pauline had a successful operation for cancer of the sigmoid colon, but the histology showed involvement of the lymph nodes in the specimen. She was therefore offered adjuvant chemotherapy with 5-FU and folinic acid injections. These were given daily, from Monday to Friday of one week every month, for a total of six months. After the first course of chemotherapy, Pauline developed mouth ulcers and diarrhoea, but after the treatment dose was reduced, she had no further side effects.

She remained completely well for the next year, but a routine CT scan then revealed a single metastasis in the liver. She was treated with further chemotherapy, comprising an infusion of 5-FU given through a Hickman line, and injections of another drug, mitomycin C. After three months of treatment, there was a substantial reduction in the size of the liver metastasis, and an MRI scan was performed to confirm that there were no other metastases present. Pauline then had an operation to remove the liver metastasis, which was successful.

After she had recovered from the operation, a further three months of chemotherapy was recommended. She has now completed this, and she remains well at present, with no evidence of active disease.

10 Support groups and counselling

If you have cancer, it is important that you know you are not alone. There are cancer support and self-help groups throughout the United Kingdom and all over the world. There are also many local groups, and information should be available from doctors' surgeries or from directories at local libraries. Moreover, do not forget the support that a local church community may be able to give.

Most large hospitals will have a patient support group, which will provide a way for you to meet other people with colorectal cancer and discuss your problems with them. Often, such groups will put out a newsletter or organise talks by specialists or professional carers working in the field. This is also a good way of learning about new treatment advances.

The following national associations will give emotional support and practical help to men and women with colorectal cancer or to their friends and relatives. The addresses given are often for a head office and there may be many branch offices. A freephone number can be used to gain information about groups in your area.

This is not an exhaustive list. In particular, the websites listed for these organisations frequently point the user towards other helpful organisations supplying additional specialist information on treatment, symptoms, patient support groups and recent research findings.

Colon Cancer Concern

Colon Cancer Concern provides a helpline for anyone who needs support or information on colon cancer. Specialist nurses may be available. The organisation carries out research and produces a regular newsletter. Fact sheets are also distributed.

Colon Cancer Concern
Department of Surgery
Chelsea and Westminster Hospital
369 Fulham Road, London SW10 9NH
Tel: 020 7381 4711 (helpline, Mon-Fri, 10am to 4pm)
Website: www.coloncancer.org.uk/home.htm

British Colostomy Association

The British Colostomy Association has a national network of over 20 area organisers, supported by small teams of trained volunteers. They provide information and support for anyone about to have a colostomy or who already has one. If you wish, you can be introduced to people who already have, or have had, a colostomy.

British Colostomy Association

15 Station Road
Reading
Berkshire RG1 1LG
Tel: 0800 328 4257 (freephone)
Email: sue@bcass.org.uk
Website: www.bcass.org.uk

Cancerlink

Cancerlink is for people with any kind of cancer, not just colorectal cancer. It is used by cancer patients, their friends and families and professionals working with them. Information is provided by telephone, email and letter.

This information service can offer support and information and help you to clarify treatment options, so that you can make a better decision. A range of booklets discussing cancer and its emotional impact are available. Cancerlink will also put you in touch with cancer support and self-help groups in your own area through the Directory of Cancer Support and Self Help.

Cancerlink

11-21 Northdown Street
London N1 9BN
Tel: 08088 080 000 (freephone)
Email: cancerlink@canlink.demon.co.uk
Asian language information and support telephone line (Hindi, Bengali, Gujerati, Punjabi, Urdu and Cantonese): 08088 080 000 (freephone)
Young people helpline: 08088 080 000 (freephone)
Note: The telephone service given above for all categories is available only on Mondays, Wednesdays and Fridays, between 10 am and 6 pm.

British Association of Cancer United Patients

The British Association of Cancer United Patients (BACUP) gives advice and information about all aspects of cancer, as well as emotional support for people affected by cancer and their families and friends. Their Cancer Information Service is staffed by a team of specially trained nurses and supported by a panel of medical specialists. BACUP's Cancer Counselling Service is available to anyone who can travel to the London office. They can also help you to find a counselling service if you live out of London.

BACUP

3 Bath Place, Rivington Street
London EC2A 3JR
Website: www.cancerbacup.org.uk
Cancer Information Service:
All areas Tel: 0808 800 1234 (freephone)

Beating Bowel Cancer

This charity, run by people who have had bowel cancer, aims to raise awareness of bowel cancer and improve every stage of a patient's journey, by informing and supporting patients and their families.

Beating Bowel Cancer

39 Crown Road, Twickenham TW1 3EJ
Tel: 020 8892 5256; Fax: 020 8892 1008
Website: www.bowelcancer.org

Cancer Care Society

The Cancer Care Society offers free counselling, emotional support and practical information, rather than medical support, to people whose lives have been touched by cancer. It has support groups run for and by people with direct experience of cancer. This society also has telephone link arrangements for individual support, arranging contact between enquirers and those in their own area with similar experiences.

Cancer Care Society

11 The Cornmarket, Romsey
Hampshire SO51 8GB
Tel: 01794 830 300; Fax: 01794 518 133
Email: info@cancercaresociety.org
Website: www.cancercaresociety.org/

Macmillan Cancer Relief

Since hospices and palliative care specialists (those who treat patients to minimise their symptoms and improve their quality of life, rather than expecting to cure the disease) have become more commonly available, especially Macmillan Cancer Care Nurses, many surgeons and oncologists have been better informed and have been able to provide more effective care for the patient, both in the hospital and in the community.

A number of Macmillan Cancer Nurses are based in hospitals and a patient can be referred by a general practitioner to such a nurse right from the point of diagnosis or at any stage of the illness. The nurse will provide emotional support, practical information and advice on an ongoing basis.

Macmillan Cancer Relief

89 Albert Embankment, London SE1 7YQ
Tel: 020 7840 7840;
Fax: 020 7540 7841
Website: www.macmillan.org.uk/
Information line: Tel: 0845 601 6161

Marie Curie Cancer Care

Marie Curie Cancer Care runs ten centres for cancer patients throughout the United Kingdom. Support is also provided in the home, by Marie Curie Nurses working together with the NHS District Nursing service.

Marie Curie Cancer Care

89 Albert Embankment, London SE1 7TP
Tel: 020 7599 7729
Fax: 020 7599 7708
Email: info@mariecurie.org.uk
Website: www.mariecurie.org.uk

Imperial Cancer Research Fund

This is primarily a research organisation but the website is worth watching for the latest trial information.

Website: www.icnet.uk/research/factsheet/bowel.html

Improving Outcomes in Colorectal Cancer

This is also primarily a research site, set up by the Department of Health.

Website: www.doh.gov.uk/canc/colrecs.htm

Tak Tent Cancer Support – Scotland

Tak Tent Cancer Support – Scotland offers information and support for cancer patients, their families and friends. There is a network of support groups across Scotland that meet monthly. A 'drop-in' resource and information centre is available. Youth projects work with patients aged 16-25 years.

Tak Tent Cancer Support – Scotland

Block C20
Western Court
100 University Place
Glasgow G12 6SQ
Tel: 0141 211 1932
Website: www.easynet.co.uk/aware/contacts/taktent/

Tenovus Cancer Information Centre (Wales)

Tenovus offers support and information on any aspect of cancer to both patients, relatives, friends and health professionals. Services are free, confidential and available in both English and Welsh. The Cardiff centre is also a drop-in centre, providing a range of leaflets, fact sheets and books. For confidential and professional advice, use our Freephone Cancer Helpline 0808 8081010.

Tenovus Cancer Information Centre (Wales)

Velindre Hospital
Whitchurch
Cardiff CF14 2TR
Tel: 029 2019 6100

The Ulster Cancer Foundation

The Ulster Cancer Foundation in Northern Ireland provides information and support for patients and relatives.

The Ulster Cancer Foundation

40-42 Eglantine Avenue, Belfast BT9 6DX
Tel: 02890 663 439
Website: www.ulstercancer.org

Colostomy Care Group, Irish Cancer Society

This Colostomy Care Group gives support to patients who are about to have or have recently had surgery to treat colorectal cancer. Specially trained volunteers, who have themselves undergone colorectal surgery, are available to discuss problems or anxieties and provide support and encouragement. Contact with patients is personal and confidential.

Irish Cancer Society

5 Northumberland Road, Dublin 4
Ireland
Tel: 01 668 1855
Fax: 01 668 7599
Email: support@irishcancer.ie
Website: www.irishcancer.ie/support/colostomy.html
Cancer helpline:
Tel: 1 800 200 700 (freephone)

Social Security benefits and legal advice

If you are diagnosed with cancer, you may qualify for extra Social Security benefits or you may need legal advice. If so, the National Association of Citizens Advice Bureaux may be able to help you. There are about 1500 bureaux nationwide and all of these can provide free, impartial, confidential advice and help. The national address is:

National Association of Citizen's Advice Bureaux
115-123 Pentonville Road
London N1 9LZ

Look in your local telephone directory for details of any local Citizens Advice Bureau.

11 The future

Surgery and chemotherapy

Scientific knowledge is increasing all the time, and new treatments are continually being developed and tested. Surgical techniques are being improved constantly. Drugs such as mitomycin C, irinotecan and oxaliplatin, at present used in advanced cancer, may have a role in the early stages as well. New drugs are under development all the time, such as eniluracil, which is intended for use with 5-FU to increase the effect of 5-FU and allow it to be taken orally.

Different methods of administering drugs are also being compared, for example a single injection versus intravenous infusion. The effects of different doses of various drugs are being tested. Moreover, the order in which drugs are given may be important.

Screening

New methods of screening are being refined and may be used more widely in the future, such as the faecal occult blood screening test (a test for unseen blood in the stool). Increased cost-effectiveness may eventually allow screening of the general population rather than selected people at risk, as at present. Molecular markers may be used to determine the presence or predict the behaviour of colorectal cancer, thus allowing more effective treatment. Such genetic screening tests may be more reliable than faecal occult blood tests. Some day, even genetic treatments may be developed.

Relapse

Identification of the characteristics that give an increased risk of relapse could help doctors to give more effective adjuvant treatment.

Keep in touch

These issues represent just some of the investigations that are under way at present. Support groups (see Chapter 10) will help you to keep up to date with new discoveries and will provide a source of knowledgeable people with whom you can discuss recent new scientific discoveries.

12 Answers to questions you may be asking yourself

I have seen small amounts of bright red blood on the toilet paper after I have wiped myself. I have not told my doctor because I am frightened that I might have cancer. What should I do?

Tell your doctor immediately. Your fears are most likely groundless. First, there is a very high chance that this symptom is caused by something less serious than cancer. Second, if by any chance it is cancer, this will probably be in the rectum, where you will have a very good chance of a complete cure, and the earlier, the better.

Is there a genetic screening test that could show whether I carry a gene for colorectal cancer?

Not yet. Since the gene for familial adenomatous polyposis is known, researchers are now working on tests to diagnose this disease before symptoms appear. Rapid advances have been made in understanding the genetic mechanisms underlying the development of other colorectal cancers also, but much work remains to be done. There is a clear need for more specific genetic, and also biological, markers that can be used in selective screening.

Will I have to have a colostomy and carry a 'bag'?

This depends entirely on where your cancer is and how far it has advanced. Only a small proportion of people with colorectal cancer need such an operation. Sometimes, the operation is only temporary. New surgical approaches mean that some patients who would previously have had an external colostomy can now avoid this inconvenience.

Does radiotherapy cause long-term damage?

Radical doses of radiotherapy used for rectal cancer do carry some long-term morbidity, particularly with bowel function and continence. Modern techniques have reduced this, but not eliminated it.

Will chemotherapy side effects ever go away?

Most side effects are short-lived, although it may not seem like that at the time. Nausea and vomiting are controlled completely or very successfully in most patients. Hair loss is by no means universal, although a wig is usually needed for a few months beyond the chemotherapy period in those who lose their hair. In women, suppression of the ovaries, by chemotherapy, may mean that menstrual periods disappear during treatment. Often, they come back, but for women in their late 30s and 40s, menopause may occur early. Chemotherapy can also cause abnormalities in children conceived during and after treatment. Therefore, fertile women will need to use contraception while undergoing chemotherapy and for at least one year afterwards.

Will becoming a vegetarian mean that I have less risk of colorectal cancer?

There is no evidence that vegetarians are less likely to develop colorectal cancer than those who eat some meat or fish. A balanced diet is very important for general health. You should eat plenty of raw fruit and vegetables each day, and you should not overbalance your diet with large amounts of protein-containing or fatty foods. High levels of alcohol are also unwise. Regular exercise, even just walking, is likely to help.

My specialist wants me to enter a clinical trial. Should I agree?

Clinical trials have advantages and disadvantages. Some of the advantages are that you may be getting the latest treatment and your progress will be very closely monitored. However, since the treatments are still at an experimental stage, you may be running risks. If the trial is a controlled, blinded one, you may receive the same treatment you are getting at present without knowing it. Your doctor is obliged to tell you about all the known risks.

Abdominoperineal excision
Surgical operation to remove a rectal tumour using combined approaches from both above and below the rectum (known as APE, APER or APR).

Adenomatous polyp
A small benign growth arising from the layer of cells lining an organ. In the colon, this is the first layer of cells (epithelium) beneath the mucous membrane. See also Polyp.

Adjuvant therapy
Additional or complementary treatment that is usually given after surgery. It may consist of chemotherapy or radiotherapy or both.

Anaemia
A disorder of the blood in which the oxygen-carrying pigment in the red cells is below normal levels. A feature of many different diseases.

Anal canal
Passage leading immediately to the anus.

Anal sphincter
The ring of muscle that guards the opening of the anus and allows a person to evacuate the rectum or hold the contents in at will.

Anorectal
Involving the anus and the rectum.

Anterior colorectal resection
Surgical removal of part of the colon or rectum by approaching through the front of the abdomen.

Anus
The opening or 'back passage' through which comparatively solid waste matter is discharged from the body.

Ascending colon

The right side of the large bowel, which ascends from the bottom of the abdomen to the top and has a high fluid content.

Ascites

Excessive collection of fluid in the abdomen, caused by secondary cancer attacking the abdominal lining. It can be drained by a tube.

Barium enema

An X-ray test of the bowel. Barium is inserted into the bowel to make the details show up better.

Benign growth

A relatively harmless swelling that does not spread into the surrounding area or to other parts of the body. A benign tumour does not recur after surgical removal.

Bile duct

Bile is a greenish-brown liquid produced by the liver. It is carried from the liver to the small intestine by the bile duct. Obstruction causes jaundice.

Biopsy

Removal of a small piece of tissue for examination by a pathologist.

Caecum

A pouch between the small bowel and the large bowel, sited just above the appendix.

Chemoradiation

Treatment with drugs plus X-rays. May be given before surgery to shrink the tumour.

Chemotherapy

Treatment of cancer using drugs.

Colitis

Inflammation of the colon.

Colectomy

Surgical removal of part or all of the colon.

Colocolonic anastomosis

Surgical operation that removes part of the colon and joins the two ends up again.

Colon

The longest stretch of the large bowel, both enables nutrients to be absorbed into the body and carries away waste matter. It rises on the right side where the contents are fairly fluid, then crosses transversely over the top of the abdomen from right to left, descends on the left side and then curves into the pelvis (sigmoid colon) to reach the rectum as the contents become more solid.

Colonoscopy

The use of a video endoscope on the end of a flexible tube to examine the large bowel.

Colostomy

An operation in which part of the colon is taken out and the remaining end is directed to an outlet on the front of the abdomen. A bag is needed to collect faeces from the outlet.

Computed tomography (CT) scan

A painless method of examining sites deep within the body.

Constipation

Infrequent or difficult passing of bowel movements.

Crohn's disease

A chronic inflammatory disease that can affect any part of the gastrointestinal system. It may cause pain, fever, diarrhoea and loss of weight.

Descending colon

The left side of the large bowel, which descends from the top of the abdomen.

Diarrhoea

Frequent passing of unusually loose bowel movements.

Dysplasia

Abnormal growth of tissues, for example as a result of long-term ulcerative colitis.

Endometrium

The lining of the womb.

Epidural anaesthetic

An anaesthetic introduced around the membrane covering the spinal cord that gives a loss of feeling below the waist.

Faeces

Bodily waste material discharged through the large bowel.

Faecal occult blood (FOB) test

A test to detect blood in the faeces that cannot be seen with the naked eye. It is expensive at present and is not wholly reliable. However, it can give an indication of whether there may be a problem and it is completely painless as it is done on a stool sample.

Familial adenomatous polyposis

A disease that runs in the family in which numerous benign polyps grow in the mucous membrane of the colon and often cause bleeding. Can lead to cancer.

Gastrograffin

A contrast medium, like barium, and used in the same way.

Genetic material, genetic mutations

Genes determine an individual's characteristics, which are inherited from previous generations. Genes are formed from deoxyribonucleic acid (DNA). Alterations in this material are called mutations. Some mutations can cause cellular malfunctions that lead to cancer.

Hartmann's procedure

A surgical procedure in cancer in which part of the sigmoid colon (or rectum) is removed, with one cut end brought out as a colostomy and the other closed and left inside the abdomen.

Haematology

Study of the blood.

Haemorrhoids

Also called piles. Swollen veins in the lining of the anus which may cause bleeding and pain.

Hemicolectomy

Surgical operation that removes half the colon (either left or right).

Hysterectomy

Removal of the womb.

Ileocolic anastomosis

Surgical operation that removes part of the colon and joins the rest to the small bowel.

Ileorectal anastomosis

Surgical removal of the entire colon, with the small bowel joined to the rectum.

Ileostomy

Surgical removal of the entire colon and rectum with the end of the small bowel brought out through the front of the abdomen. A bag on the outside of the abdomen is needed to collect the waste.

Intestine

This is the major part of the digestive system and extends from the exit of the stomach to the anus. It is situated below the stomach and occupies much of the central and lower parts of the abdomen. It forms a long tube with two large sections, the small intestine (small bowel) and the large intestine (large bowel or colon). The function of the intestine is to break down and absorb food and water into the bloodstream and to carry away the waste products of digestion.

Intravenous infusion

Delivery of drugs directly into a vein through a catheter or tube over several hours or days. With a continuous line, the infusion may last for several months.

Irritable bowel syndrome

A combination of intermittent abdominal pain and irregular bowel habits (intermittent constipation or diarrhoea) in the absence of a diagnosed disease. It is not life-threatening but can cause great distress.

Jaundice

Yellow colour in the skin and eyes caused by liver damage or blockage of the bile duct. Can be caused by metastatic colorectal cancer.

J pouch

A pouch made from the end of the small bowel, in order to provide some of the reservoir function lost when the rectum is removed.

Lymph, lymph nodes, lymphatic system, lymph vessels

Lymph is a colourless fluid containing white blood cells, proteins and fats. It is carried around the body in a network of minute vessels or tubes called the lymphatic system. It absorbs fats from the intestine in particular. Lymph nodes are small organs lying at quite frequent intervals along the course of a lymph vessel. They vary considerably in size, from microscopic to about 2.5 cm in diameter, and can act as a barrier to the spread of infection by destroying or filtering out bacteria.

Malignant tumour

A swelling made up of abnormal cells that have the ability to spread into the surrounding tissues and to other parts of the body.

Magnetic resonance imaging (MRI)

A painless method of diagnosis that scans sites deep within the body.

Mesentery

A sheet of tissue containing the bowel's lymphatic nodes, through which malignant cells can spread.

Mesorectum

The mesentery of the rectum.

Metastases

Secondary tumours that develop when cancer cells invade blood vessels or lymph channels near the site of origin (the primary site) and are carried to other parts of the body.

Metastasectomy

Surgery to remove a metastasis.

Mucosa

The colon is lined with a membrane composed of mucosal cells.

Mucosal dysplasia

A disorder in the size, shape, rate of multiplication of mucosal cells.

Mucosectomy

Surgical removal of the lining of the top of the anal canal.

Oncologist

A doctor who specialises in the treatment of cancer.

Orthopaedic operation

An operation involving bone.

Ovaries

In women, produce reproductive cells (eggs). One ovary is situated each side of the womb in the lower abdomen.

Palliative treatment

Treatment that is designed to delay a relapse and relieve the symptoms of the disease rather than to cure it.

Panproctocolectomy

A surgical operation to remove the rectum and colon and close up the anus permanently. A bag is needed on the front of the abdomen to collect waste.

Pathologist

A specialist who uses a microscope to examine cells removed by biopsy in order to determine whether a tumour is benign or malignant.

Pelvis

A basin-shaped cavity surrounded by bone at the lower end of the torso or body trunk.

Perineum

The region of the body between the anus and the sexual organs (scrotum in men or vulva in women).

Peritoneum

The membrane lining the cavity of the abdomen.

Platelet

The smallest type of blood cell, which is necessary for blood clotting. A platelet deficiency can cause bleeding disorders.

Pleural cavity, pleural effusion

The pleural cavity is the space around the lungs. Pleural effusion is an accumulation of fluid in this cavity, which may be caused by metastatic colorectal cancer. The fluid can be drained.

Polyp

A small growth protruding from a mucous membrane. A polyp in the colon, which is lined with this type of membrane, is considered to be an early sign that cancer may develop. It is not a cancer in itself. It can be removed by colonoscopy.

Proctocolectomy

A surgical operation to remove the rectum and colon.

Prognosis

Forecast of the likely course of the disease by an expert, based on experience with other patients.

Prostate gland

In men, a gland surrounding the neck of the bladder which releases a fluid forming part of the semen.

Radiotherapy

Treatment using radiation, often given after surgery to help remove any remaining cancer cells.

Rectum

The final, pocket-like section of the large bowel which leads into the anus.

Regional chemotherapy

Administration of drugs directly into the affected organ, often used when the liver has to be treated.

Resect, resection

A surgical term, meaning to take a piece of the colon or rectum out and then join the rest up.

Sacrum

A triangular bone near the base of the spine, situated between the two hip bones.

Secondary cancer

Cancer that has spread to another part of the body not directly connected to the original cancer site.

Segmental resection

Surgical removal of a relatively small part of the colon containing a tumour.

Seminal vesicles

In men, hold the reproductive fluid and are situated just in front of the rectum.

Sigmoid colon

The last section of the large bowel which hangs down into the pelvis and leads directly to the rectum. A sigmoid colectomy is the surgical removal of this part.

Sigmoidoscope, sigmoidoscopy

A viewing tube, either flexible or rigid, that can be introduced into the rectum and the sigmoid colon to examine the walls for abnormalities. The instrument is able to pump air into the bowel to allow a better view. It is uncomfortable rather than painful.

Stent

A plastic tube used in drainage.

Stoma

An opening. In bowel surgery, this is an artificial opening produced when a cut end of the bowel is brought out onto the skin of the abdomen. The bowel contents are drained through this stoma into a disposable bag.

Stool

A discharge of waste matter from the large bowel.

Stricture

A narrowing that may cause poor function.

Systemic treatment

Treatment of the whole body rather than therapy to the affected area only.

Total mesorectal excision

Surgical removal of the mesorectum, a membrane containing lymph nodes that surrounds the rectum, together with the rectum itself.

Transanal resection

Surgical operation in which the surgeon reaches through the anus to reach a cancer in the rectum.

Transanal endoscopic microsurgery

A system that allows a surgeon to operate, using binocular magnification, through a distended rectum to cut out a section of cancerous bowel.

Transverse colectomy

Surgical removal of the transverse colon.

Tumour

A swelling caused by an abnormal cell multiplying to produce millions of cells that form a lump.

Ulcerative colitis

Severe inflammation of the intestine causing ulcers to develop, which may bleed. Also causes diarrhoea. Can lead to cancer if untreated.

Uterus

The womb.

Index